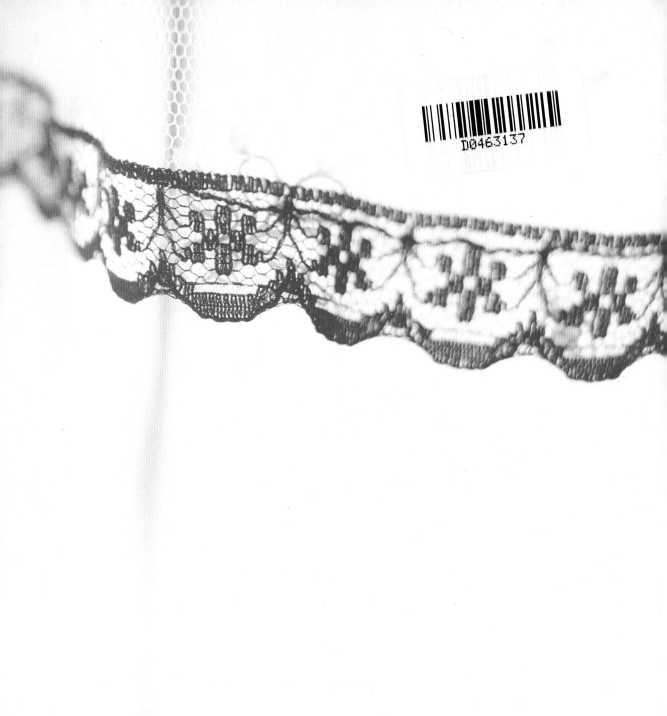

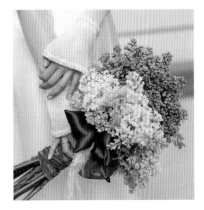

HOW TO BE A

beautiful
bride

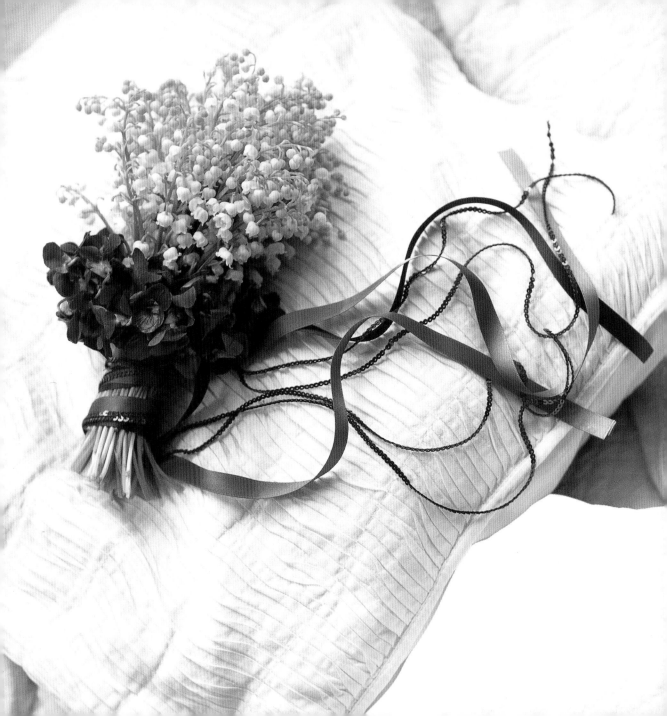

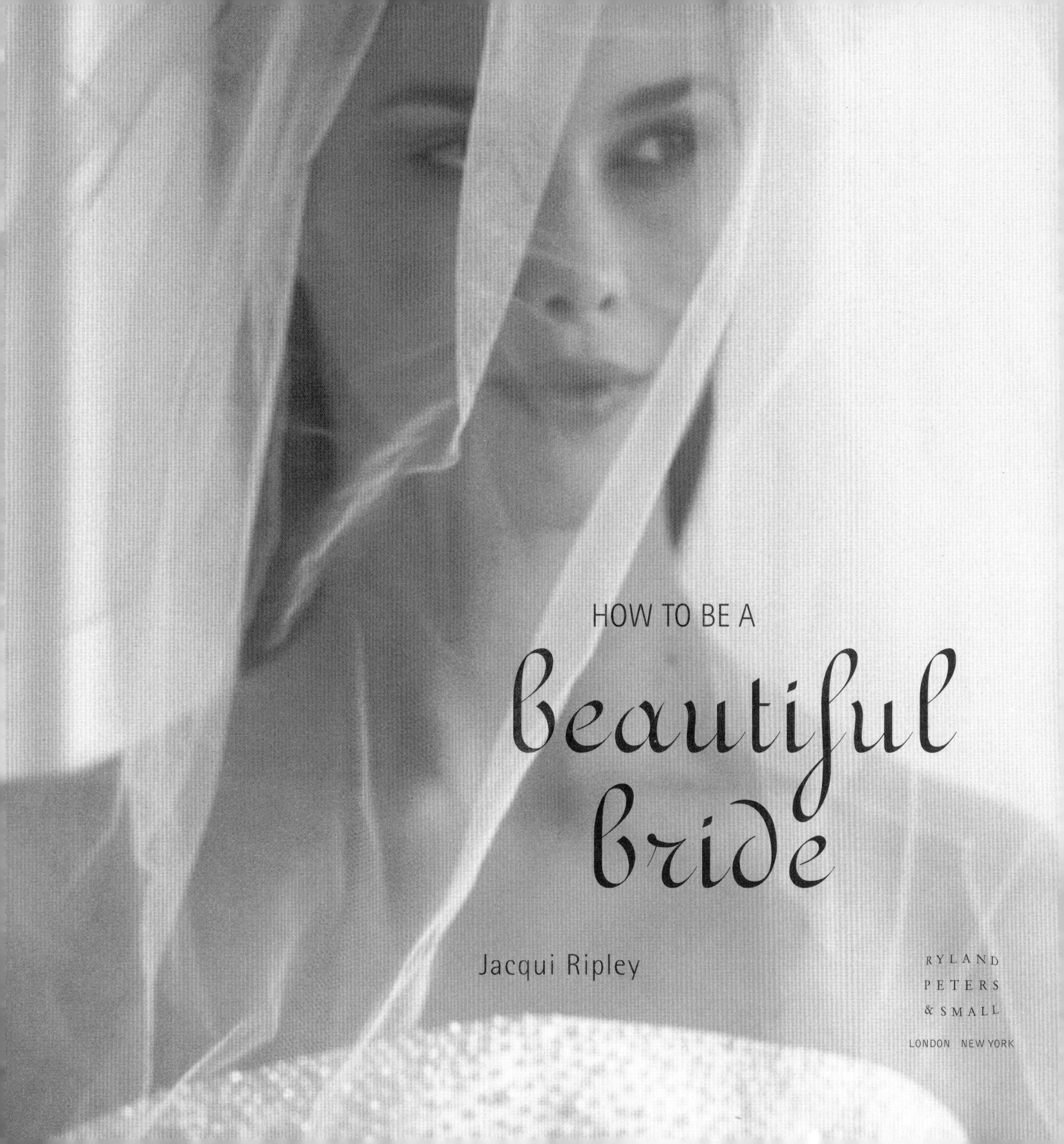

HOW TO BE A

beautiful

bride

Jacqui Ripley

RYLAND
PETERS
& SMALL

LONDON NEW YORK

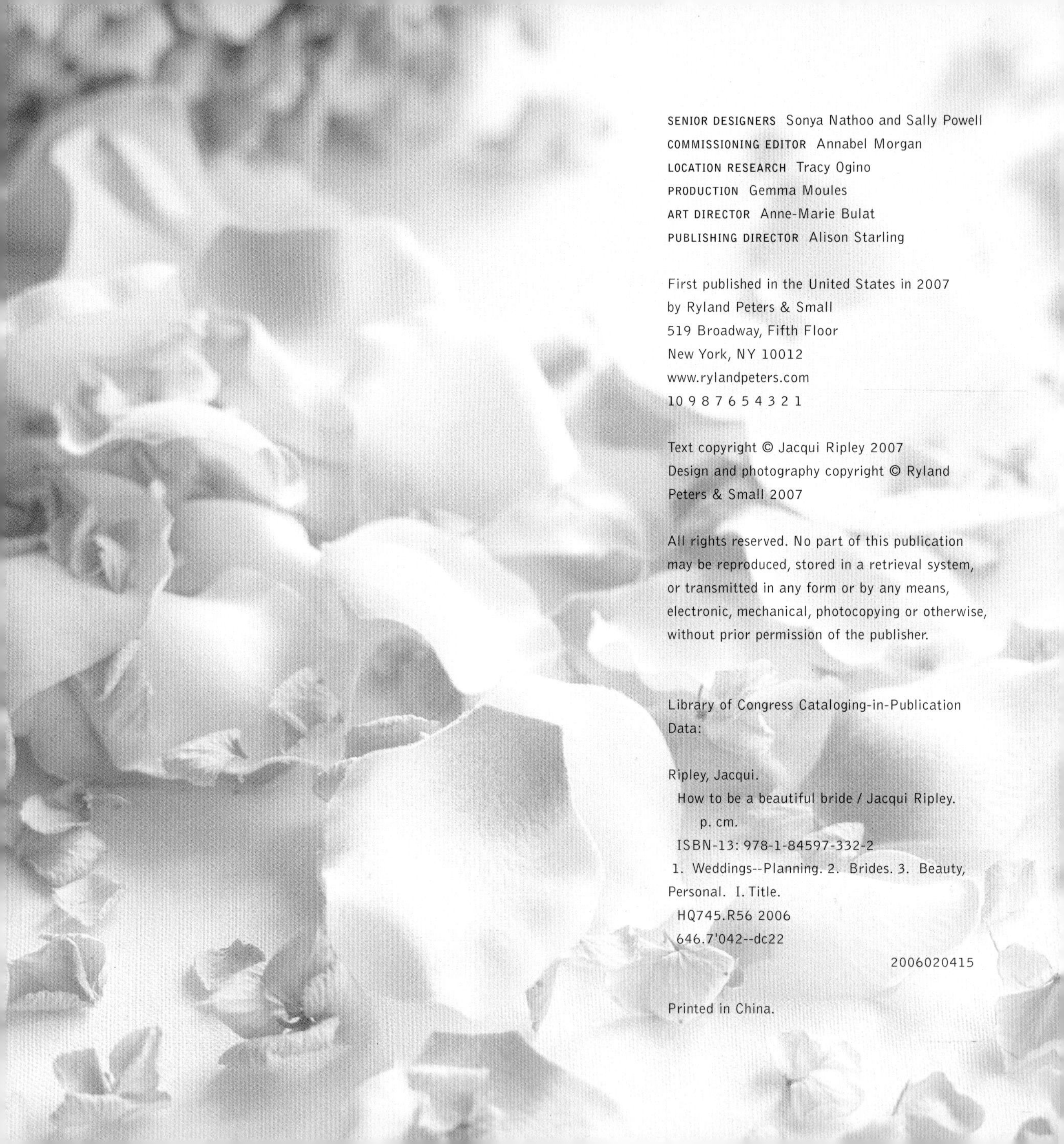

SENIOR DESIGNERS Sonya Nathoo and Sally Powell
COMMISSIONING EDITOR Annabel Morgan
LOCATION RESEARCH Tracy Ogino
PRODUCTION Gemma Moules
ART DIRECTOR Anne-Marie Bulat
PUBLISHING DIRECTOR Alison Starling

First published in the United States in 2007
by Ryland Peters & Small
519 Broadway, Fifth Floor
New York, NY 10012
www.rylandpeters.com
10 9 8 7 6 5 4 3 2 1

Library of Congress Cataloging-in-Publication
Data:

Ripley, Jacqui.
  How to be a beautiful bride / Jacqui Ripley.
    p. cm.
  ISBN-13: 978-1-84597-332-2
  1. Weddings--Planning. 2. Brides. 3. Beauty,
Personal. I. Title.
  HQ745.R56 2006
  646.7'042--dc22
                                    2006020415

Printed in China.

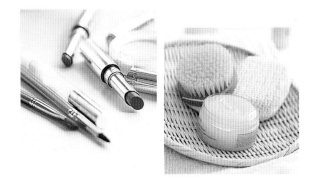

contents

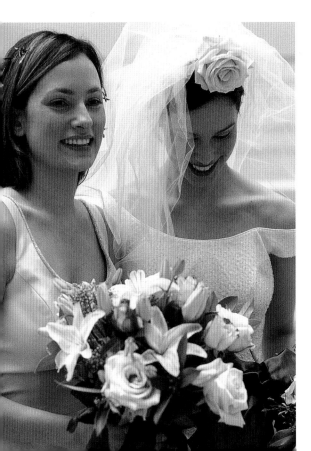

introduction

Planning a wedding is fun, exciting, and stressful all at the same time. But the most important factor for the bride is making sure she steals the limelight on her big day. Every bride wants to treasure magical memories of her wedding day forever—and for her look to be timeless. Finding your dream dress, planning your hair and make-up, getting started on figure-fixing exercises, and choosing accessories are among a bride's top priorities.

If you're stressing over all these details, relax. Within these pages are many inspired ideas you'll love, along with expert tips to ensure that you'll look and feel beautiful and to help you radiate an aura of serenity and happiness on your big day.

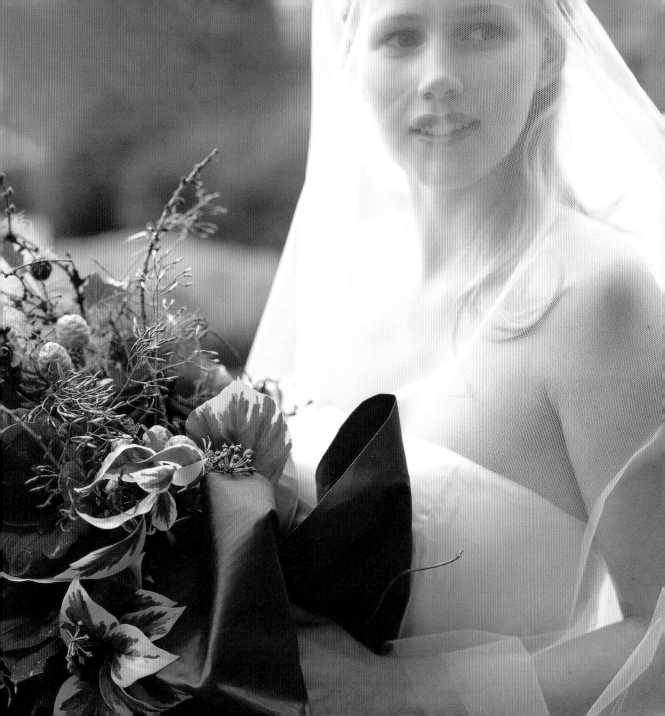

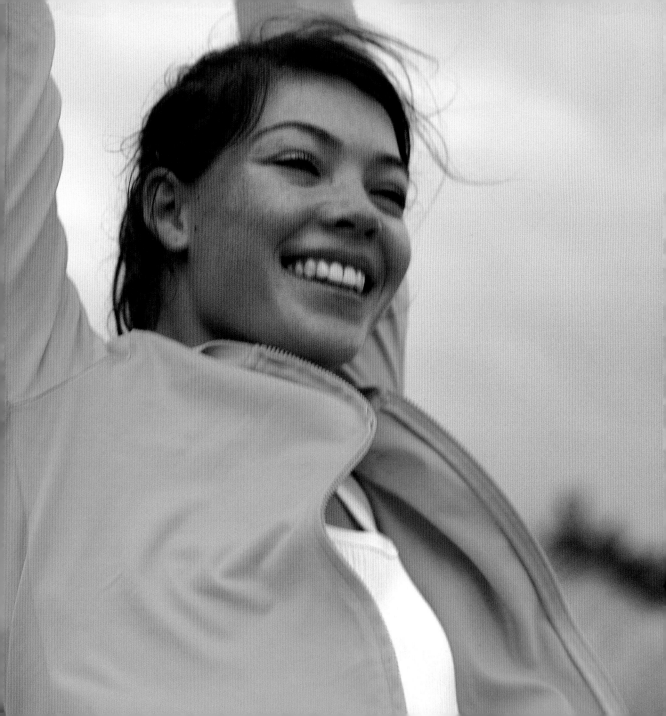

getting in shape

Being tight, toned, and flab-free isn't as hard as you think. The trick to looking fabulous in your wedding gown is to tackle any problem areas by using troubleshooting exercises that will shape and define your figure.

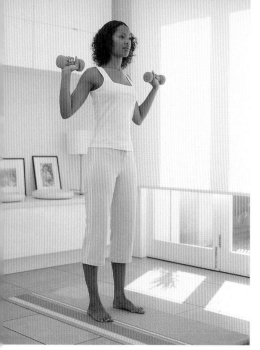

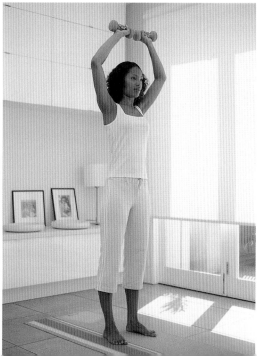

shoulders and bust

Hitting the gym to get fit and firm on top of organizing one of the biggest days of your life can seem too much to take on. But focusing on improving your problem areas will keep your fitness plan realistic and do-able.

SHOULDER TONER

This exercise gives your shoulders definition—ideal if your dress is strappy or strapless. It's easy to overlook shoulders, but by defining them you keep your arms looking great, too.

1 Stand with your feet shoulder-width apart, your tummy pulled in, and shoulders back and down. Hold a 3–5 lb dumbbell in each hand with palms facing out. Keep arms bent at 90 degrees and weights held at shoulder level.

2 Press dumbbells straight up, lifting your arms overhead. Keep arms as close to your ears as possible while raising your arms into an arch.

3 Lower the weights to the starting position. Rest for a moment, then repeat the exercise. Start with one set of 10, increasing to three sets of 15.

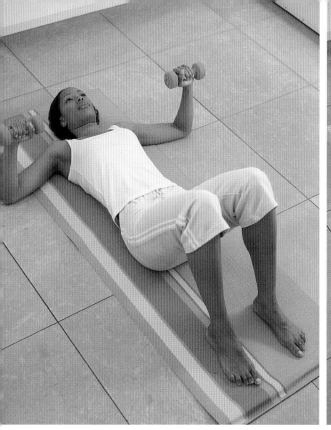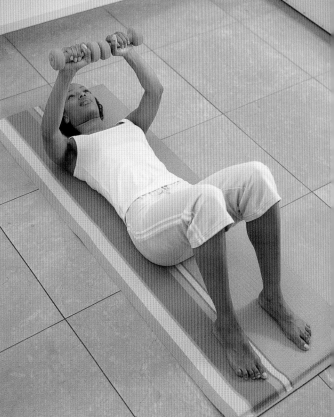

BUST FIRMER

Unfortunately, exercises cannot increase the size of your bust, but they can strengthen and tone the surrounding pectoral muscles (the underlying muscles around the breasts), giving you a better lift.

1 Lie back on the floor with knees bent, holding a dumbbell in each hand. Keep elbows bent at 90 degrees and the upper arms resting on the floor.

2 Slowly press hands straight up and bring weights together over your chest (not your head). Lower arms back down to the starting position. Rest and repeat. Start with one set of 10, increasing to three sets of 15.

• Palm presses are a great no-fuss bust-boosting exercise. Press your palms together under your chin and in front of your bust, as if praying. Hold for a few seconds, relax, and then repeat 20 times.

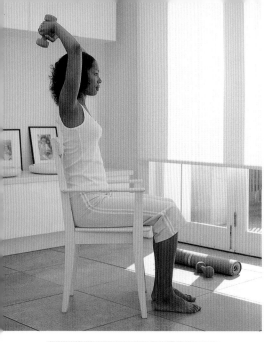

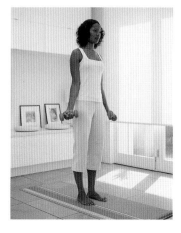

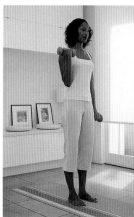

arm shapers

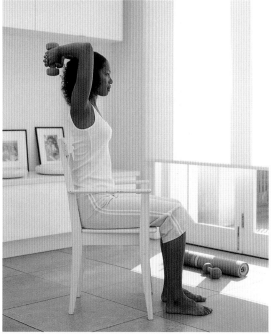

For toned arms, your triceps and biceps (as well as the upper back) need to be worked out. The secret is to imagine yourself in a slinky sleeveless top—that should send you running for the dumbbells!

FOR THE TRICEPS (LEFT)

1 Sit on a chair, with head up, back straight, and feet on the floor. Hold one dumbbell vertical to the floor with both hands overhead.

2 Keeping your upper arms in place, slowly lower the dumbbell straight down behind your head as low as you can comfortably go, keeping elbows at one fixed point.

3 Lift the dumbbell back up over your head until arms are fully extended. Start with one set of 10, slowly increasing to three sets of 15.

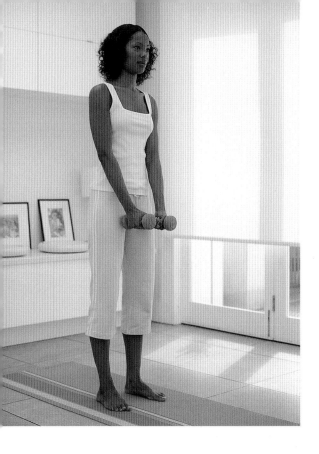

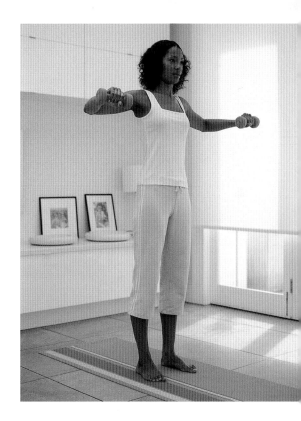

FOR THE BICEPS (ABOVE LEFT)

1 Stand with feet shoulder-width apart and arms by your sides, holding a dumbbell in each hand.

2 Leaving your left arm relaxed and pointing to the floor, slowly bend your right arm up to a 45-degree angle and continue to bring the weight right up to your shoulder. Lower until the arm is straight.

3 Repeat with the opposite arm. Aim for three sets of 10–15 reps per arm.

FOR THE UPPER BACK (ABOVE)

1 Stand with feet hip-width apart and a dumbbell in each hand, palms facing in, and arms in front of the body. Keep elbows relaxed and tummy pulled in.

2 Slowly lift your arms out to the side, keeping elbows relaxed. Your elbows should be bent at 90 degrees and parallel to the floor. Lift your arms no higher than shoulder level. Hold for a couple of seconds, then lower. Start with one set of 10, increasing to three sets of 15.

tummy toners

WAISTING AWAY

A defined waist gives any figure better proportion. Frequent abdominal workouts can transform your figure from shapeless to hourglass.

WAIST STRENGTHENER (BELOW)

1 Lie on your side and place your elbow under your shoulder for support. Place one foot on top of the other and pull in your tummy muscles.
2 Slowly lift yourself up, using your obliques (waist muscles) to keep the position. Lift your arm over and above your head. Hold for a count of 10–20 seconds. Repeat on the other side.

TWIST CRUNCHES

Lie with knees bent and feet flat on the ground. Place your hands under your head with elbows out to the side. Keeping hips still, slowly turn the upper body to your right, so the upper back and shoulders come off the floor. Lower, and repeat on the other side.

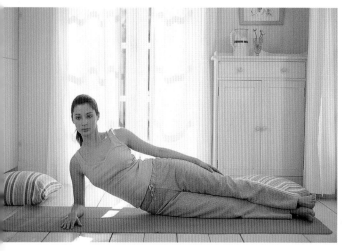
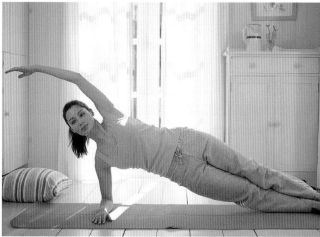

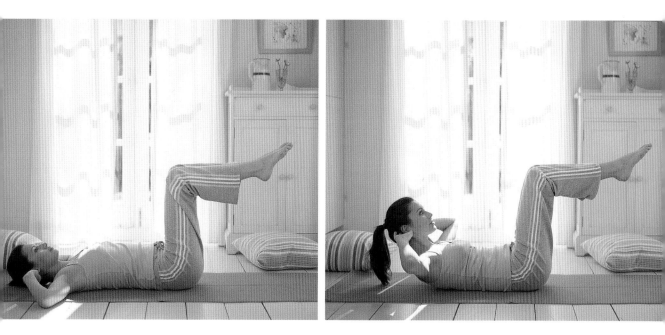

STOMACH SMOOTHERS

A flatter stomach gives you added confidence, and helps to support your back and improve your posture.

MID-AB CRUNCH (ABOVE)

1 Lie flat on your back with arms at your sides and legs raised in the air at a 90-degree angle to your body.
2 Push your lower back firmly into the floor and lift your upper body with your hands behind your head, crunching upwards. Do two sets of 30 reps.

LOWER-AB CRUNCH (RIGHT)

1 Lie on your back with hands under your butt. This will tilt the pelvis up slightly and support the lower back.
2 Lift your legs up and bend your knees almost to a 90-degree angle. Lift your pelvis and butt back towards your ribcage. Aim for two sets of 30 reps.

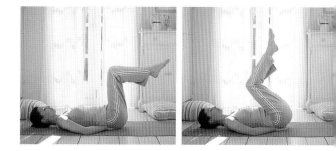

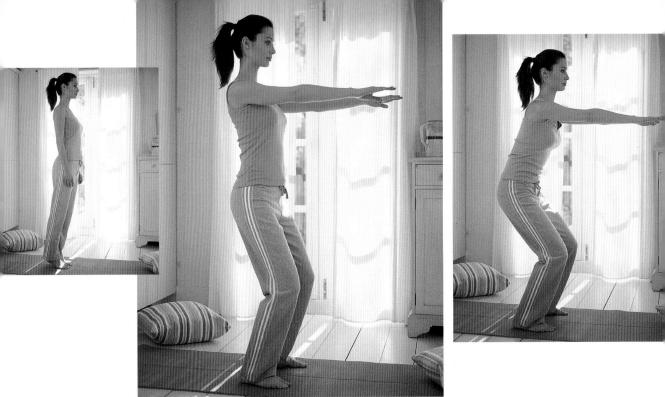

butt and legs

THIGH AND BOOTY BOOSTERS
Exercise can help your butt and thighs tone up quickly, giving you a more streamlined shape.

SQUATS (ABOVE)
1 Stand with feet shoulder-width apart, toes turned out and knees slightly bent.

2 Slowly lower yourself into a squat (as if sitting down) until your knees are directly above your ankles. Return to starting position. Repeat 15 times for three sets.

BUTT CLENCHES
When sitting or standing, squeeze and clench your glutes for five seconds, then release. Repeat 20 times.

THIGH TRIMMER (BELOW)

1 Lie on your right side, with head, shoulders, and hips aligned. Support your head with your right hand and place your left arm in front of you for stability. Bend your left leg and place it in front of your right leg.

2 Keeping your right leg straight and foot flexed, slowly lift your right leg about 6–8 inches off the ground. Keep your leg lifted for a second at the top of the movement, then lower. Repeat for 8–12 reps for three sets. Repeat on the other side.

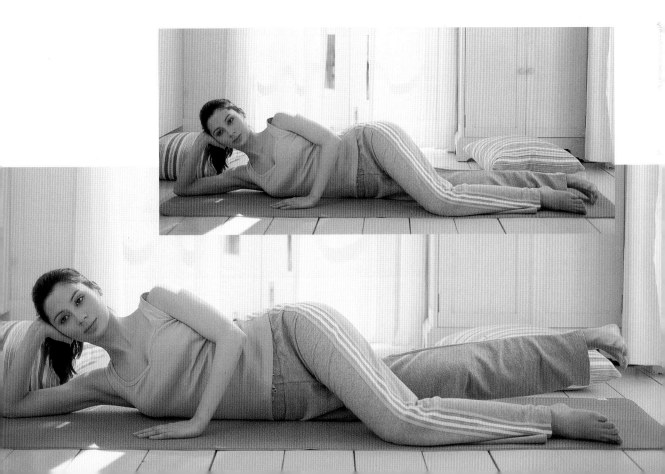

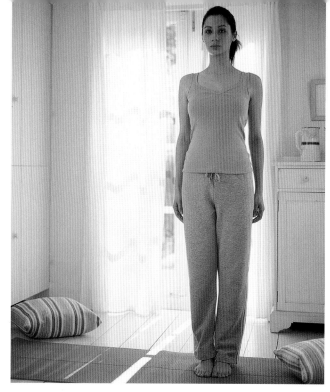

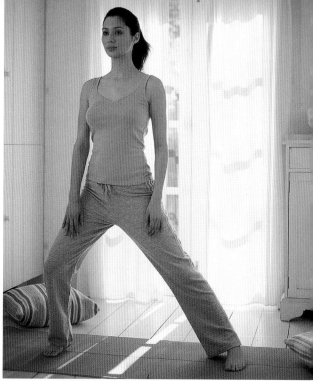

LEG SLIMMER (ABOVE)

Walking is a great way to exercise your legs, but you can also slot in a few targeted moves if you want to tone them faster.

1 Stand tall, feet together, toes facing forward. Take a wide step to the right with your right foot and bend your right knee, so you're in a side lunge.

2 Place your hands just above your right knee, hold for one second, then squeeze your butt and return to the starting position. Hold, then lunge again. Repeat for 15 reps on each side for three sets.

CALF SHAPER

1 Stand with feet together, toes facing forward and arms by your sides. Lift your heels and roll onto the balls of the feet. Hold for a second, then lower. Repeat 20 times.

WALL SQUATS

Stand two feet away from a wall with arms by your sides. Sit back, as if onto a chair, until your back is flat against the wall and your thighs are parallel to the floor. Hold this position until your legs get tired, then lower yourself to the floor. Repeat up to 10 times.

a class act to follow

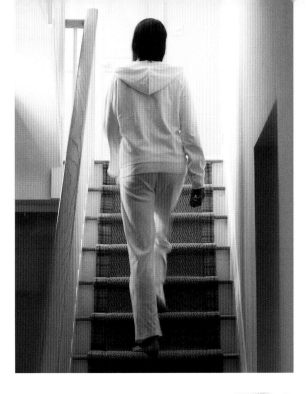

To help take your figure from average to amazing, why not try a class to stretch, tone and burn off calories?

PILATES A slow and precise form of exercise that helps you achieve body awareness. Helps lengthen and strengthen muscles, as well as improving posture and rebalancing the body.

YOGA Ancient healing form of exercise that can improve energy, increase flexibility, build strength, center your emotions, and induce a sense of calm. Start off with relaxing Hatha yoga or, if you want something more challenging, try the aerobic-style Ashtanga.

AEROBICS A fantastic way to get fit while having fun. Covers all the body bases, from stretching through to conditioning and cardiovascular work.

BELLY DANCING Lots of fun, as well as a great ab workout. The deep abdominal muscles and pelvic floor are worked, and belly dancing also shapes and sculpts the waist, hips, and thighs.

EASY MOVES

☆ *Take the stairs for an all-over butt and leg shaper. Take two at a time for better results.*

☆ *Crank up some tunes and dance. Your body will thank you for it.*

☆ *Walk in heels. It trains your legs to produce muscle, especially in the calves and thighs.*

☆ *Focus on pulling your abs back toward your spine at all times. You'll target the deep abdominal muscles that are responsible for keeping your tummy taut.*

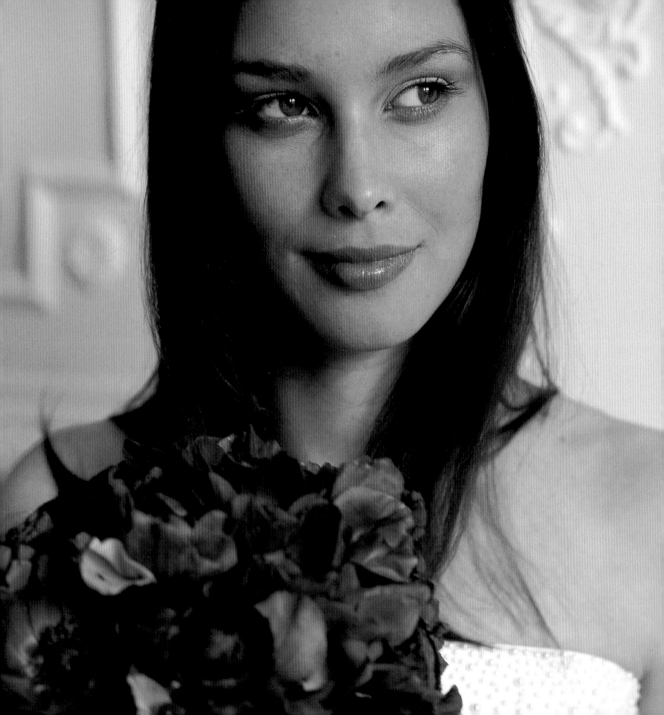

getting gorgeous

Great skin, strong nails, glossy hair—ever thought there might be a connection? Good nutrition is the foundation for all these things, and eating the right foods is one of the hardest-working beauty treatments.

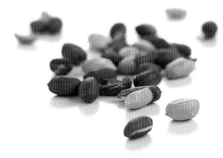

becoming a beauty gourmet

"ACE IT" Great skin requires vitamins A, C, and E (also known as antioxidants). They protect skin from free-radical damage. Beta-carotene is found in brightly colored vegetables and fruits, and is converted by the body into vitamin A, which prevents dry skin. Vitamin C plays a leading role in the production of collagen and is found in meat, fish, and eggs. Vitamin E is present in eggs, avocado, sunflower seeds, and whole-wheat bread, and ensures better use of oxygen by the skin cells.

EAT FISH A couple of portions of fish a week will help keep hair nourished and glossy and nails strong. Sardines, salmon, and mackerel all contain omega-3 fatty acids, which are essential for beauty maintenance.

ZOOM IN ON ZINC Increase your zinc intake, as skin, nails, and hair feed off this nutrient. You'll find it in nuts, seeds, wheatgerm, and poultry.

PACK IN PROTEIN Hair is a protein, nails are made up of layers of a protein called keratin, and skin cells can't repair themselves without sufficient amounts of protein. Amino acids are the building blocks of protein, and are found in meat, poultry, fish, eggs, nuts, pulses, and beans.

DETOXIFYING DRINKS Sip dandelion tea to help cleanse the kidneys and liver. Drink a cup three times a day to help your body get rid of waste products and detox stressed skin.

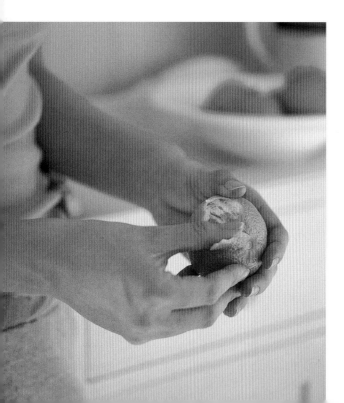

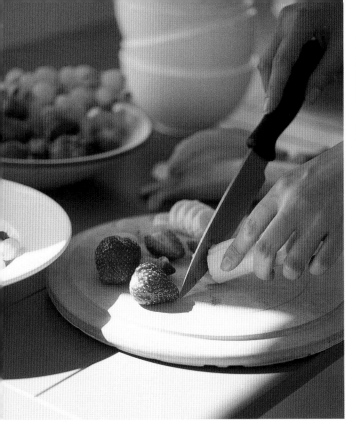

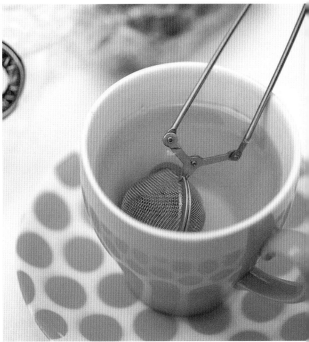

ENERGY FOODS TO GO Use food as an energizer to bring a healthy glow to your skin.

• Pick the right fruit. Apples, pears, and berries take some time to digest, so they therefore provide more sustained energy.

• Fill yourself with beans. Baked beans, kidney beans, chickpeas, and lentils are top energy foods.

• Avoid fast foods. Too many processed foods make skin dull and hair listless. Eat foods that are as fresh as possible.

SUPPLEMENT SMART

A varied diet should address all your nutritional and beauty needs, but the following minerals are often lacking from women's diets:

☆ *Magnesium. Helps to repair and maintain body cells. Important for strong teeth. RDA 300mg.*

☆ *Iron. A deficiency shows in brittle nails, hair loss, and lack of energy. RDA 14mg.*

☆ *Zinc. Essential for cell repair. RDA 15mg.*

skin spoilers

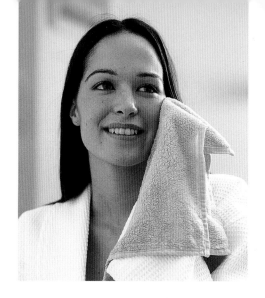

Falling into bad lifestyle habits can affect the way your skin looks and functions. Experts now believe that changing the following bad habits can benefit the overall appearance of your skin.

TOO MUCH ALCOHOL Alcohol constricts the blood vessels and dehydrates the skin, giving it a dry, weather-beaten look. Alcohol robs your skins of essential vitamins and nutrients, and impairs liver function. If the liver isn't flushing out toxins sufficiently, the skin will appear sallow.

TOO LITTLE WATER The difference between the look of a grape and a raisin is water! Insufficient water intake can result in a spotty and lackluster complexion. Did you know that one caffeinated drink robs the equivalent of four glasses of moisture from your body? Try to drink 8–10 glasses of water a day. Carrying a water bottle around with you will help you meet this quota.

SMOKING You don't even have to be a smoker for your skin to suffer from this nasty habit. A passive smoker's skin is at risk, too. In addition to the increased likelihood of premature aging, smoking starves the skin of oxygen and reduces its ability to generate collagen. Nicotine also deprives the skin of essential nutrients; especially vitamins A and C.

YO-YO DIETING An endless cycle of weight gain and loss stretches the skin to the point of no return, and this is where elasticity drops significantly. A healthy weight drop is up to two pounds a week. Any more than that and you will be losing lean muscle tissue, which is when the face can start to look gaunt.

EXCESS SUGAR In recent years, our sugar intake has risen at an alarming rate. When there's too much sugar in your bloodstream, the excess sticks to protein fibers between your skin cells, causing premature aging. To beat sugar cravings, be sure to eat little and often, and combine protein-rich foods with carbohydrates.

FOODS THAT BEAUTIFY

☆ *Avocado. A skin treat rich in vitamin E, which is essential for healthy eyes.*

☆ *Beetroot. A rich source of iron, vitamin A, vitamin C, and calcium. Also contains other nutrients that are excellent for the skin and strengthen blood vessels.*

☆ *Blueberries. A "superfood" with blood-cleansing properties. A good source of vitamins and minerals.*

☆ *Grapes. Boast polyphenols—power antioxidants. They aid in digestion, speed up the detox process, and help improve your skin.*

☆ *Carrots. A good all-rounder, high in fibre, vitamin C, and beta-carotene.*

☆ *Lemons. Great body cleansers with essential bioflavonoids and twice as much vitamin C as oranges. Slice into hot water and sip instead of tea or coffee.*

skin fitness

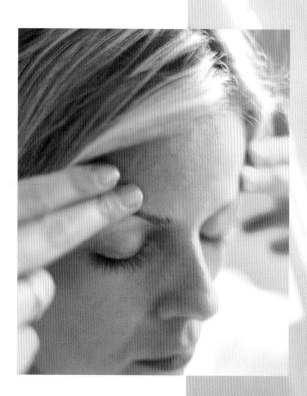

For a flawless complexion, it's essential to adopt a good fitness routine for your skin in the months leading up to your wedding. Perform facial exercises and massage in addition to following an effective skincare regime.

FACIAL WORKOUTS Holistic experts believe facial exercises give a natural face-lift and restore radiance. While facials will unblock pores, it's the supportive facial muscles that keep skin firm. Exercises help give these muscles a workout as well as resulting in improved collagen production in the deep skin tissues.

JAW FIRMER Sit upright and tilt your head back toward the ceiling. Keeping your lips closed, start a chewing motion. You will feel the muscles working in your neck and jaw area. Repeat 20 times.

EYE TONER Press two fingers on each side of your temples while opening and closing your eyes quickly. Repeat up to 10 times.

FOREHEAD SMOOTHER Draw your eyebrows down over your eyes. Wrinkle your nose up as far as possible. Hold for a count of 10, relax, and repeat five times.

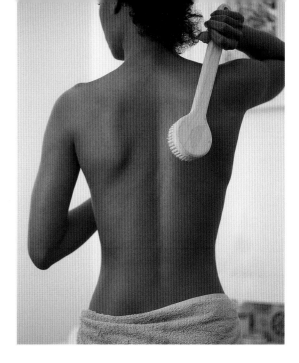

FEEL-GOOD MASSAGE Massage stimulates blood flow, drains toxins, and relaxes the skin. Face tapping is a good place to start. Make light, quick taps with the pads of your middle fingers all over your face, then use your palms to make sweeping upward movements using a favorite facial moisturizer.

SKIN STRATEGIES Lay down skin commandments in your quest for gorgeous skin. Cleansing, moisturizing, and exfoliating are fundamental to daily care. Skin problems crop up when dirt and dead skin cells aren't removed. Good skin relies on moisturizing, which hydrates skin cells, leaving skin plump and healthy.

ALL AGLOW Exfoliation brightens your complexion. A twice-weekly scrub will help control breakouts, alleviate dryness and minimize the appearance of fine lines. Two ingredients that have been scientifically proven to result in radiant skin are alpha-hydroxyl acids and retinols. Look for them in moisturizers and night creams.

BLEMISH FIGHTERS High levels of the stress hormone cortisol and adrenaline cause acne. Don't rely on it to clear up by itself—see your doctor to ask about antibiotics months before your wedding. Use products that are non-comedogenic and contain salicylic acid, which unclogs pores and gets rid of dead skin cells.

SKIN TIPS

☆ *Energize eyes by applying a light eye cream with your ring finger before bed.*

☆ *Use a facial mask while bathing. Steam opens pores and encourages deeper penetration.*

☆ *Sun damage is the top reason skin appears dull. Wear moisturizer with an SPF and fake your glow.*

☆ *To treat a new blemish, wrap an ice cube in muslin and hold to the spot. This will take down the swelling, making it easy to hide with concealer.*

body gloss

For a smoother, sleeker body, capture some all-over skin radiance with these brilliant bare-it-all tips.

GLEAM ON An all-over scrub will remove dead cells from the skin's surface, leaving it soft and more receptive to moisture. Exfoliate with a body brush from the feet up before showering, or use a scrub. Pay attention to less obvious areas, such as ankles, knees, elbows, and the back of arms. These are places where dead cells build up, leaving skin thick and dull. If you find the back hard to reach, use a towel. Hold one end over your shoulder and the other down by your opposite hip, then slowly rub back and forth slowly. Switch sides to make sure you've exfoliated your entire back.

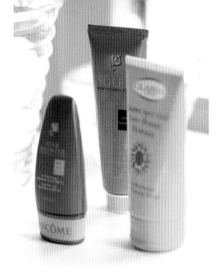

MUST-HAVE MOISTURE Adequate moisture will leave skin looking supple, with a more even skin tone. When using body products, remember that they need to work at a deeper level, so it takes longer for results to show. Start applying the body cream early for visible results on your wedding day. For maximum moisturizing, don't apply body lotion right after bathing. Wait until your skin is completely dry. Otherwise, it ends up absorbing moisture too quickly.

THE BUZZ ON FUZZ Hair removal is an essential beauty chore. Stubbly or hairy underarms and legs don't make for a great photo opportunity! Hair removal should be done before applying fake tan—tanning lotion can get trapped around short hairs and give a spotty finish. If you decided to shave, be sure your blade is new, and use shaving foam to prevent any nicks. Waxing and cream depilatories make for a satiny smooth finish (wax at least two days before your wedding to allow skin to recover). Prevent ingrown hairs by exfoliating the legs and applying tea-tree cream.

SUN-KISSED SKIN A fake tan warms up skin, evens out imperfections and makes you look slimmer. Pulling off a natural color is all in the application. Apply the tan two nights before the wedding, to avoid stains on your dress and to allow the color to fully develop. First exfoliate, then dry and moisturize your body. Start at your feet and work your way up, applying self-tanner on one section of your body at a time. Smooth over skin with long, vertical strokes, followed by horizontal ones, until the cream is completely absorbed. Use less cream on your joints, where color can collect in creases. Use a separate product for the face and apply from the center of the face outward. Blend at the jawline and around the ears. Keep cream away from the hairline and eyebrows.

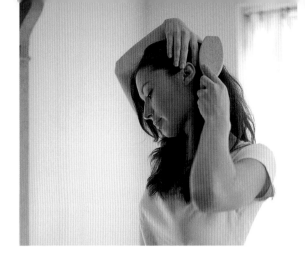

getting hair happy

Most brides have an idea of how they want their hair to look on their wedding day, but you also need to think about the condition, cut, and color of your tresses.

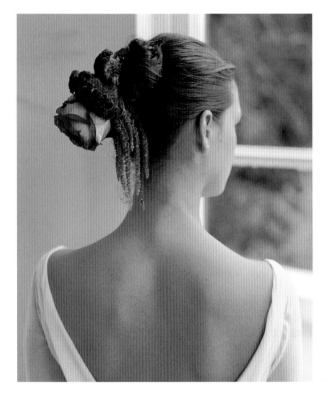

HIGH–CLASS HAIR Washing your hair is the single most important aspect of hair health. Shampooing stimulates the hair follicles, and hair should look its best when it is freshly washed. If it doesn't, you're either using the wrong products or not shampooing correctly. For a foolproof technique, apply shampoo, gently massage the scalp for about a minute, then rinse thoroughly.

CLEVER CONDITIONING Follow shampoo with the correct conditioner for your hair type. Pay extra attention to the ends—they're always drier. If hair feels rough, look to creamier formulas or invest in an intensive conditioning mask.

A CUT ABOVE THE REST Good-hair days start with a great cut. Visit your hairstylist at least six months before the big day for a consultation. If you need to grow out your bangs or old color, this will give you time. It's also the right time to experiment with new styles. If you're thinking of changing your style, bring a along a picture of what you want. A picture is worth a thousand words! If your hair has been damaged by chemicals or over-processing, your locks could be full of split ends. The only cure is to snip them off. Half an inch off the ends every six weeks will result in healthier hair.

TUNE INTO COLOR Great color freshens up your hairstyle, injects volume, and boosts shine. Get your hair colored at least two weeks before your wedding to give it time to settle. A good colorist will give their client plenty of advice before applying color. Whether you choose to get subtle highlights or a full-on transformation, you need to consider your skin tone.

COLOR TIPS
• Warm up pale skin with honey blonde, reddish gold, or warm brown tones.
• Olive-skinned beauties should opt for auburn, amber, and caramel shades. Avoid anything bleached or brassy.
• If you have yellow skin, keep your base color dark, and highlight with lighter toffee browns. Anything too blonde will wash you out.
• Dark brown skin looks best with deep mahogany or chestnut browns, which give hair richness and depth.

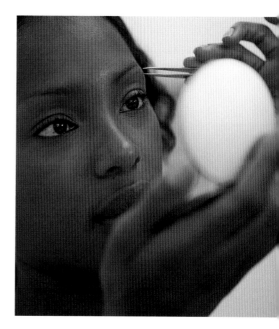

...DON'T FORGET EYEBROWS
☆ *Eyebrows frame your face, and playing around with your hair color can alter the balance of your features.*
☆ *Only tint your eyebrows darker if you have chosen a darker hair color.*
☆ *If going a lot lighter than your natural hair color, brows should be lightened slightly.*
☆ *You can use a cream bleach to lighten eyebrows or an eyelash dyeing kit to darken them, but unless you really know what you're doing it's a job best left to the beauty experts!*

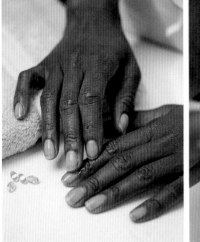
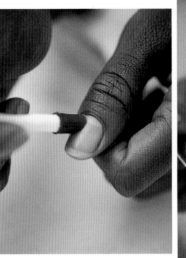
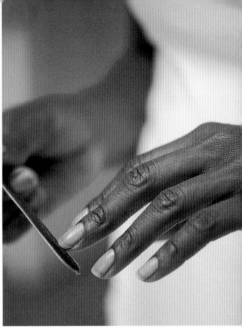

Details that make a difference

When it comes to understated but elegant bridal style, grooming is key. Subtle touches to hands, nails, and feet will bring a look together.

HANDS-ON BEAUTY

Holding the bouquet, exhanging rings, and greeting guests makes a bride's hands very important on the big day. You want hands to look great, so start wearing rubber gloves when gardening or doing household chores. Like your face, give hands a "facial" by exfoliating and moisturizing regularly. When applying a face mask, put some on the backs of the hands as well.

PRETTY AND POLISHED

If you're a chronic nail biter, start booking weekly manicures or do them yourself. It gets you into the habit of having pretty, groomed nails. Another tip is to wear brightly colored nail polish. When your nails get near your mouth, the color will catch your eye, and hopefully you'll stop nibbling! To keep your nails looking slick, file them into a "squoval" shape (neither square nor round). Try not to pick things up with your nails—use the pads of your fingers instead. And when it comes to choosing polish, stick to sophisticated shades like nude, beige, or pale pink.

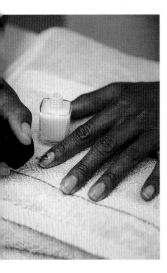

CUTE CUTICLES

For polish to look good, your cuticles need to be in excellent shape. Get into the habit of applying a cuticle oil around your cuticles before bed every night. This ensures dry skin won't ruin the look of your manicure. For instant conditioning, break open a vitamin E capsule and massage the oil into the cuticles. Massaging the nail bed with the base of your thumb brings the blood to the surface, which stimulates growth.

THE FOOTSIE LOW-DOWN

Even if you're not wearing open-toed shoes, bridal feet should still be buffed and polished. The skin on the foot is unique, as it's four times thicker than anywhere else on the body. Calluses are a common problem. Get rid of these hard areas of built-up dry skin by buffing the heels and sides of the foot with a pumice stone twice a week. Always dry feet properly; moist areas are a breeding ground for fungal infections. Apply foot cream and cuticle oil at night before bedtime to give the moisture a chance to soak in.

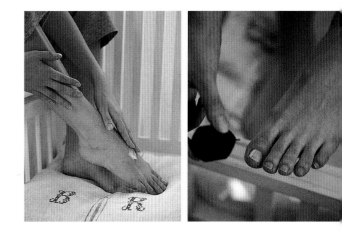

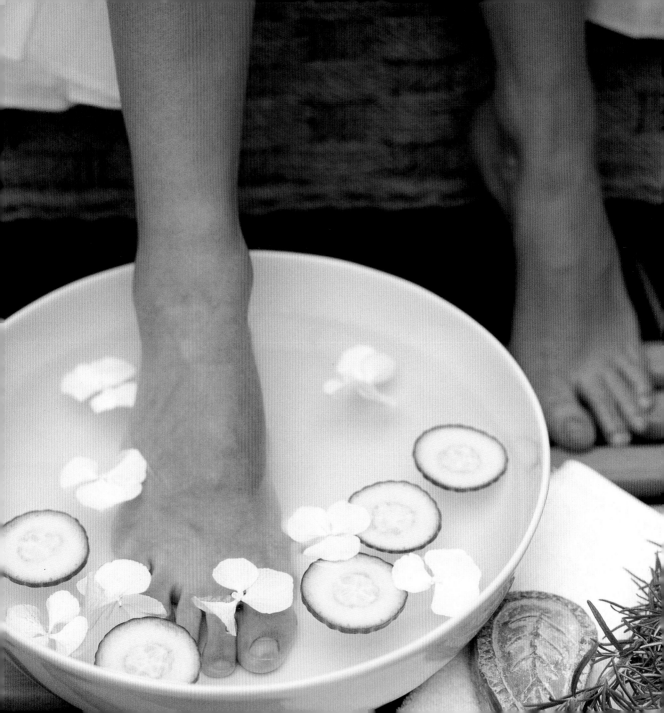

home treatments

Beyond doing pedicures, manicures, and self-tanning at home, consider indulging in a few alternative beauty treatments that benefit not only the way you look, but also how you feel.

from spa to home

Bring the spa experience right into your home with deluxe beauty treatments to protect and pamper. Sometimes skin demands a little TLC, especially if you're stressed, so look to a skin-saving solution with a freshly made mask. After a soothing facial steam (add lavender or chamomile oils), apply the following:

HEAVENLY HONEY FACE MASK

A soothing moisturizing mask for plump, soft skin.

2 tsps honey

2 tsps aloe vera gel

1 vitamin E capsule

Mix together the honey and aloe vera gel. Break open the vitamin E capsule and add to the mixture. Blend then apply to a freshly cleansed face. Leave on for 10 minutes and then rinse off.

THE ULTIMATE HAND AND FOOT TREAT

This mask will soften even the roughest of skin. You can apply it to elbows and knees, too.

1 avocado, finely mashed

1 egg yolk

1 tsp honey

3 tsps oat bran

5 drops evening primrose oil

Mix all the ingredients together, blending well, and gently massage onto hands and feet. Leave on for 10 minutes and then rinse.

BODY GLOW BLEND

An all-natural scrub is a luxury spa specialty.

1 cup fine sea salt

1 cup jojoba oil

2 drops eucalyptus essential oil

Mix all the ingredients together in a bowl. Dampen skin under the shower, then take a handful of the salt and oil mixture and massage into your skin. Rinse away with warm water.

LIP SLICK-ON

A super-kissable lip balm for pure seduction!

2 tsps beeswax

2 tsps almond oil

Heat water in a saucepan. Then place the beeswax into a bowl and set on top of the pan. Mix the oil into the melted wax. Leave to cool in a small pot or tin.

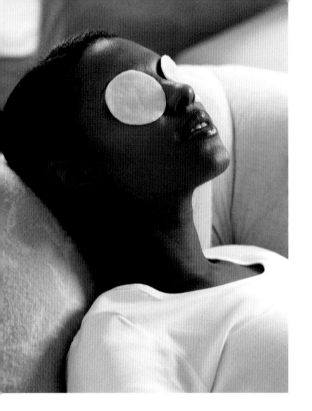

ALTERNATIVE TIPS

☆ Give yourself a good foot rub and concentrate on your solar plexus. You'll find it just below the ball of the foot. Press with your thumb to help balance the nervous system.

☆ For a bright-eyed appearance, soak two cotton pads in lukewarm green tea and then place over the eyes. Green tea is a natural anti-inflammatory and will help reduce puffiness in the eye area.

☆ Drink lots of water after any treatments, as your body has been detoxing.

STAR SPA TIPS

• The night before your wedding, apply a lifting and firming mask to your neck and chest, for a natural lift.

• Before starting a treatment, warm up a terry robe by running it through the dryer. Post-treatment, you can snuggle up in it.

• Take time out to massage in moisture. A firm stroking technique will stimulate the lymphatic system, which removes toxins and waste from your cells.

• In preparation for being on your feet all day, strengthen your arches by running them over a rolling pin.

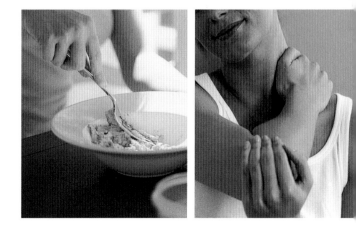

heading off pre-wedding stress

Organizing a wedding can be chaotic, so soothe your
senses, relax your mind, and find an escape with these
tension-melting ideas.

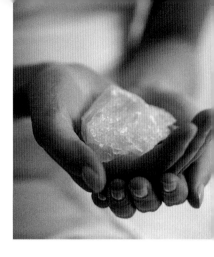

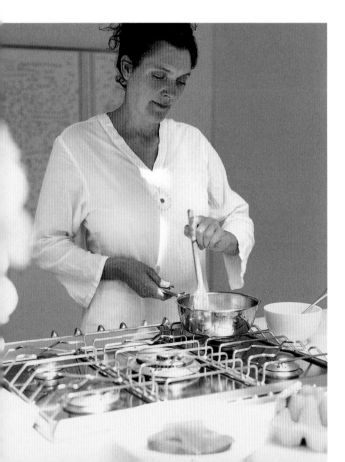

GOOD EATS Brown rice, sweet potatoes, and pasta all
contain serotonin—a relaxing chemical that calms your
mood. Munch on bananas, too. They contain vitamin B6,
which builds serotonin levels. If you're on the pill, you
could be depleting your body of this vitamin.

SPINAL SUSPENSION This is a stress-relieving pose that
rids stress from the body. Find space and hang down like
a rag doll over your thighs. Keep your knees soft. This
pose is great for releasing trapped tension from the hips,
shoulders and neck. It also brings a fresh supply of
oxygen-rich blood to the brain for improved memory
and concentration.

REACH A QUIET HIGH Deep breathing has been
scientifically proven to lower blood pressure. Next time a
situation is stressing you out, breathe out the stress. Sit
with your back straight and chest relaxed. Breathe in,
filling your lungs as much as you can. Release the air

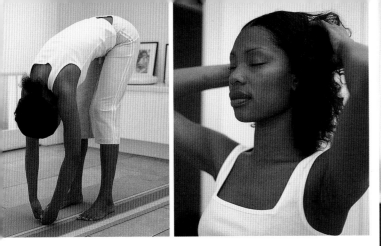

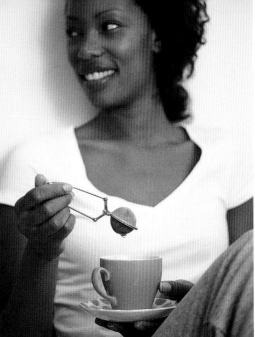

through your mouth, silently repeating "I feel calm, I feel calm." Repeat three times until tranquil.

COLOR YOURSELF CALM Wear green. In terms of color therapy, it's the colour of new beginnings, it has a positive effect on the immune system, and it promotes harmony in the body.

DON'T SAY A WORD! Give up talking. Although it may sound antisocial, "verbal fasting" is a way to find a moment of respite. Disciplining yourself to remain silent for a certain period is a great way to cleanse your mind, ground yourself, and prioritize your thoughts.

NO NEWS IS GOOD NEWS If you wake up feeling tense, avoid listening to the news. People under stress internalize bad news, so hearing about famine or war may exacerbate any worries you already have. Put on some relaxing, slow-tempo music instead.

FROM FRAZZLED TO RELAXED

☆ *Use the 24-hour rule and sleep on big decisions. It doesn't matter who is hassling you for answers—wait a day, and then reply.*

☆ *Sip lemon balm tea. It increases feelings of serenity.*

☆ *Get intimate with your hubby-to-be! Touch slows the output of the stress hormone cortisol, while giving a surge of feel-good brain chemicals.*

☆ *Appeal to your sense of smell. According to aromachology (the study of how fragrance affects moods), rose is perceived as relaxing. Spritz a rose-filled fragrance to restore a sense of peace.*

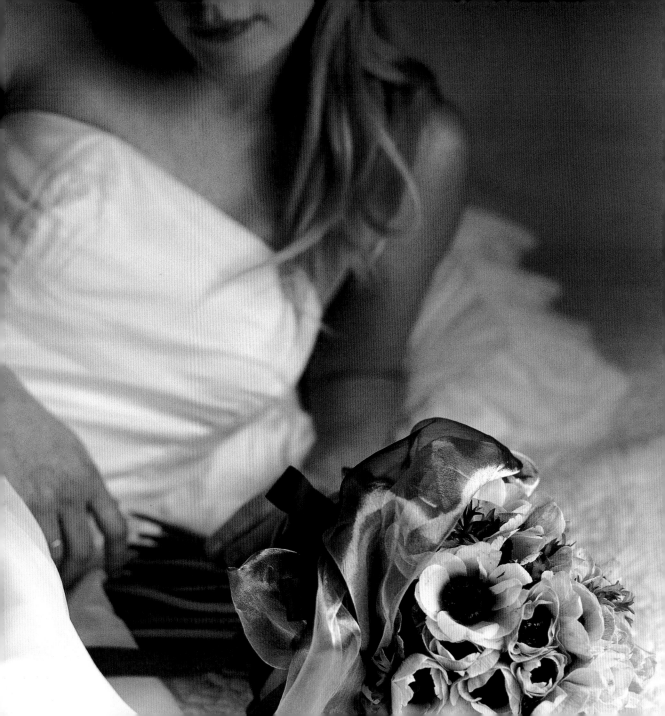

perfect bride

You've got the perfect man... Now all you want is to be the perfect-looking bride. With insider secrets on choosing the right gown, the low-down on figure-enhancing lingerie, and clever tips for hair and make-up, it's never been so easy to look beautiful all day long!

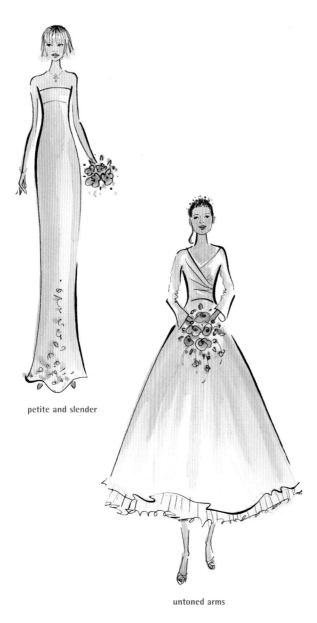

petite and slender

untoned arms

choosing your bridal-gown style

Your wedding dress has a lot to live up to, as guests will be buzzing with excitement to see it. The perfect dress will accentuate your assets and minimize any flaws. It will also give you confidence, as well as being comfortable to wear and utterly gorgeous!

PETITE AND SLENDER Empire-line dresses have a seam just below the bust and fall away to the floor. It's a style that suits slim and smaller-busted women. A column dress with a high neck is also a style that can be pulled off by those blessed with a slight figure. Steer clear of ball gowns, which can drown a petite figure.

UNTONED ARMS If you feel self-conscious about your arms, then don't show them. Either opt for a dress with full sleeves, or choose a sleeveless dress, but cover your arms with a pretty jacket, shrug, or wrap for a hint of movie-star glamour.

HOURGLASS FIGURE Consider a halter-neck gown, which gives the illusion of extending the shoulder line

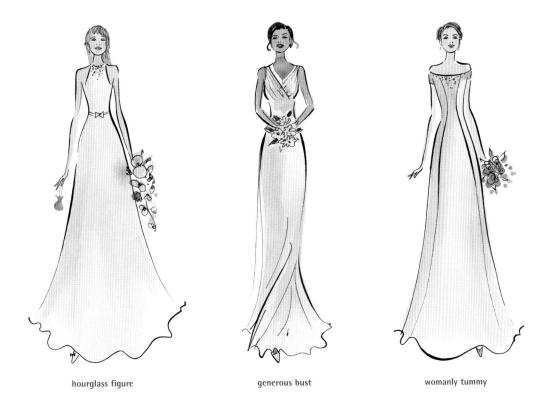

hourglass figure   generous bust   womanly tummy

and balancing out the lower body. A two piece works well if your bust is smaller than your hips. A bodice married with a ballerina-style skirt gives the figure a better proportion. Avoid straight or bias-cut designs, which only magnify the hips and bottom.

GENEROUS BUST A strapless gown can look bewitching on a curvy figure, but you will need some extra support in the bust area (see Undercover Secrets, pages 44–45). A V-shaped or scooped neckline (not too plunging) is also flattering. Avoid high necklines, which make breasts appear larger.

WOMANLY TUMMY An A-line gown is perfect. This style flares out from the waist and hides a multitude of sins! Many A-line dresses have vertical seams running from the top of the dress to the bottom, so there are no seams across the dress at the tummy area. Leave the beading to the upper part of your dress. Avoid bows or sashes around the waist, as they will only add bulk.

choosing your bridal-gown style   **43**

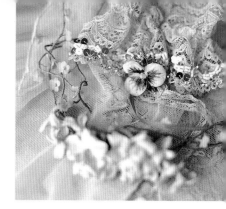

undercover secrets

Lingerie should be much more than an afterthought. The right underwear gives the hidden support you need to make your figure look better and your dress look amazing. Just as you should choose a dress to flatter your shape, so you should also choose underwear to suit the style of your dress—think of it as a fail-safe foundation. Buy your wedding lingerie before you start your dress fittings, as it may alter your shape slightly.

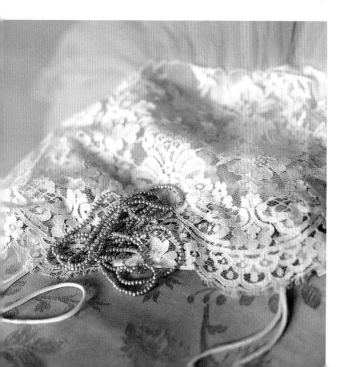

FIGURE-SKIMMING SILHOUETTE First off, check the color of your bra under the dress—it should be completely invisible. Consider seamless underwear, which makes for super-smooth foundations.

BOLD AND LOW-BACKED Unless you're very small breasted, don't think you won't need support for a strapless gown. Go for an adhesive bra. Shop around for different styles to suit your dress. The support is less than that of a regular bra, but they will hold the breasts in place, provide coverage, and give some shape.

SWEET AND STRAPLESS Strapless bras are ideal for strappy or low-cut dresses. Why not sew your bra into the dress? It will give you extra support and ensure the dress doesn't slide down and cause a revealing moment!

GENEROUS FIGURE Tackle trouble spots with control underwear, also known as shapewear. Hold-you-in basques, pants and bras are an easy route to a cinched-in waist, higher bottom, or flatter tummy.

QUICK-FIX LINGERIE TIPS

☆ *Thongs can be unflattering in a bottom-skimming dress. If a visible panty line is a problem, try a French-cut panty, which offers high-cut legs.*

☆ *For a small-breasted boost, tuck gel pads into your bra. For a bigger boost, slip on a gel-filled underwire bra.*

☆ *For a plunging neckline, look for a double-stick adhesive bra. Place it under the breasts, then lift them to create cleavage. Because it's sticky on the front as well, it allows you to fix your dress in place for extra confidence.*

☆ *To avoid nipple show-through if wearing a sheer bra, stick on a couple of nipple covers. These fabric discs offer a non-peekaboo smooth look!*

☆ *Don't buy a bra without trying it on. Weight loss or gain will alter the size of your boobs!*

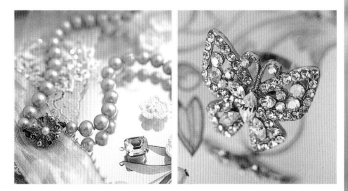

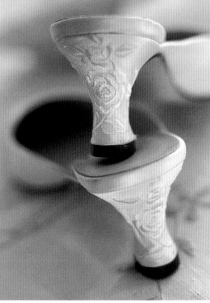

luxury bits and pieces

Just like the dress, your wedding accessories should be planned and thought out with care. Accessorizing with style adds glamour and panache to your whole look.

JEWELRY It may be tempting to wear Grandma's diamond earrings, the bracelet your mother bought you, and a pendant your fiance gave you, but if you don't want to look overdone, opt for just a couple of pieces. Match any stones found in your dress or headpiece with those in the jewels you choose. Pearls will complement beading, whereas diamonds go well with sequins or crystals. Let your hairstyle and headpiece dictate the earrings. Bejeweled drop earrings look great with an upswept do, while studs won't steal the fanfare from a decorative headpiece.

HAIR ACCESSORIES The headpiece you choose will depend on whether your hair is long or short, or whether you are wearing it up or down. Like your jewelry, your style of headpiece will reflect your personality—keep it low-key or go for something elaborate. Once only seen on the heads of society brides, tiaras are now worn by many modern brides. Decorative headbands in the fabric of your dress can look great, as can jeweled combs. Feathers and flowers can be used either in a headpiece or woven into the hair.

GLOVES AND SHRUGS If you opt for gloves, match the color to your wedding dress, and pair simple gloves with decorative dresses, or more elaborate gloves with a simple gown. As for length, wear a glove that ends just below or above the elbow with a short-sleeved dress, an "opera" glove (to just below the armpit) with a strapless gown, and wrist-length gloves with a long-sleeved dress. Remove gloves just before the ceremony, wear them for formal photographs, and take them off when eating! Ask your dress designer about cover-ups. A long tailored coat, bolero, pashmina, or a shrug are all good choices.

SHOES Wedding shoes need to look elegant as well as be comfortable. The height of your shoes is important. If you're not relaxed in high heels, your wedding is not the best time to wear them! Consider lower kitten heels or a ballet slipper, which look very pretty with a ballerina-length gown. Don't feel restricted to "wedding" shoes, either—go beyond bridal and shop around.

FRAGRANCE Fragrance has a powerful effect on memory, so you want to wear a scent that will make your heart skip a beat whenever you smell it again. If you're thinking about wearing a different "wedding" scent, leave yourself time to sniff out something new. Don't forget to ask your partner if he likes your choice! Weddings are full of emotions and the body heat that's generated will intensify any fragrance, so keep that in mind before wearing a strong scent. Consider the seasons, too. A fresh floral scent is perfect in spring and summer, whereas a heavy exotic scent would be more suitable in fall or winter.

ACCESSORY TIPS

• If you choose flowers for your hair, talk to your florist about the best types to use. You need robust blooms rather than ones that wilt quickly.

• If you have a hand-tied bouquet, ask the florist to wind the ribbon all the way down the stems. You don't want them snagging your dress or gloves.

• Try on wedding shoes at the end of the day, when your feet are at their largest.

• Make sure there's a large umbrella in the wedding car, just in case it rains.

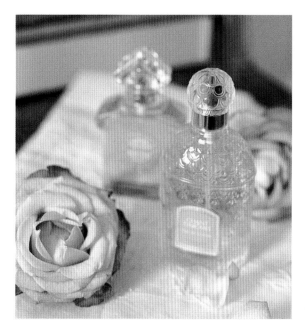

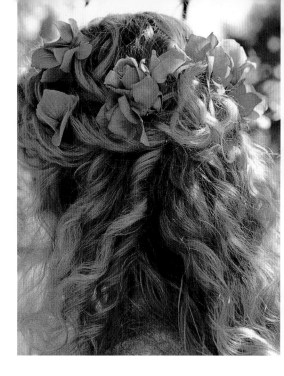

a head-turning affair

Now that the condition of your hair is enhanced with good nutrition, and the texture and shine improved with good products, it's time to find the perfect hairstyle.

BEFRIEND YOUR STYLIST Three months before the wedding is a good time to start discussing ideas with your stylist. Take along pictures of looks you like, so they can advise on what style will suit your face shape. If you want your stylist to do your hair on your wedding day, book them early and make sure they are totally happy with the date. There's nothing worse than having a stylist cancel at the last minute.

THE TRIAL RUN Once you have booked your stylist and chosen your headpiece, make an appointment with your stylist around two weeks before your wedding day, to try out the various looks. Let them know the style of your dress, as it will dictate how you wear your hair.

A STYLE TO SUIT YOU Whether you want to sweep your hair up into an elegant chignon or wear it flowing down your back, your face shape is an important factor to take into account. There are a few general rules on choosing a style to flatter your face.

LONG FACE

• Hair pulled back from the face will only elongate the face further. It's flattering to have a few wispy strands tumbling down from the crown and in front of the ears.

• Avoid styles that sit on top of the head. Instead, opt for buns on the back of the head, as this will balance out your features.

• If you're wearing your hair down, do not part in the middle. Go for a side part.

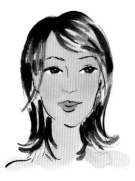

long face

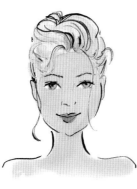

round face

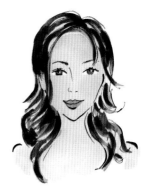

heart shape face

ROUND FACE

- Longer hair strands falling around the face give the illusion that your face is longer and slimmer.
- Loose curls piled on top of the head or a relaxed up-do will give the effect of a more shapely face. They will also add extra height for anyone wanting to appear taller.

HEART SHAPE

- Inject some fullness into the bottom half of your face with falling tendrils and waves that finish at the chin. This will also make a large forehead seem less broad.

GOING TO GREAT LENGTHS Of course, the length of your hair will have some influence when it comes to choosing the right style. There's no point yearning for a particular style if your hair just isn't long enough!

LONG HAIR There are endless ways to wear long hair. You can pile it up into a classic chignon, making a great base for your chosen headpiece.

MEDIUM-LENGTH HAIR If you want to put your hair up but are worried there's not enough length, ask your stylist about a hair sponge. These are doughnut-shaped pieces of sponge that come in colors to match your hair shade. They're placed on the crown, and hair is pinned around them. This tricks the eye into thinking you actually have more hair than you have. Low ponytails at the nape of the neck can also look stylish.

SHORT HAIR Short hair relies on a good cut. From then on, either keep your style simple or dress it up. Try a diamanté headband, a tiara, or tiny crystal hairclips.

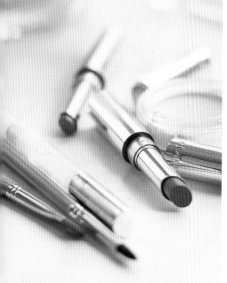

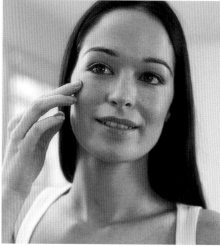

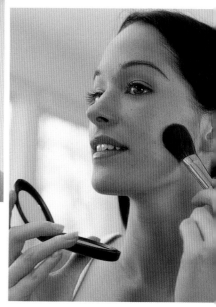

lovely make-up

On your wedding day, subtly applied make-up is essential and will help bring out the star in you.

EXPERT HELP The secret to great make-up is keeping it simple, along with a little know-how on what products to choose and how to use them. This is where a professional make-up artist comes in. If you are having your make-up applied professionally on the day of your wedding, meet up a few weeks beforehand to discuss your look, and to have a trial run before the big day. When looking for a make-up artist, word of mouth is your best option. If no one offers up names, ask around.

DO-IT-YOURSELF If you are doing your own make-up, head for your nearest department store cosmetic counters and ask about a bridal consultation. You'll be shown some professional techniques, as well as hues to suit your skin tone. This should make you more confident about applying your make-up on the big day.

FLAWLESS COMPLEXION Apply a primer before applying foundation. It forms an invisible barrier between your skin and make-up, so foundation stays put. You don't want a heavy-looking base, so keep it light, choosing a foundation that covers any blemishes

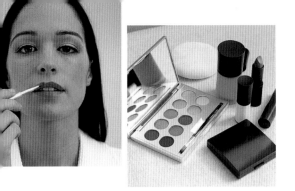

but also allows the skin to breathe. Blend foundation out and away from your nose. Cover any blemishes with a concealer that matches your skin tone. Finish with a light dusting of translucent powder.

PRETTY CHEEKS A flush of color on the cheeks makes for a pretty and youthful look. Blend a cream blush from your cheekbones up to your temples. Swirl over a dusting of powder blush to help the blush last all day.

INCREDIBLE EYES Prep the eyelids with eyeshadow primer or face powder to help color stay put. Play it safe by brushing just one shade over the lid, from lashes to crease. Resist the temptation to go for brightly colored hues. If you want to use something more exciting than taupe—sparkly gold powder, perhaps—apply the eyeshadow with a dampened brush. This makes for a less glittery and more shimmery feel. Run an eye pencil close to the roots of your upper lashes, then smudge the outer corners. Curl your eyelashes and apply two coats of waterproof mascara.

LUSCIOUS LIPS Kissing, eating, and sipping champagne can take its toll on your lipstick, so either wear a long-lasting formula, or line and fill the mouth with a neutral lip pencil for extra staying power. Keep in mind that shades close to your own lip color are low-maintenance and can be reapplied quickly. A dramatic red can look striking but will need frequent touch-ups.

MAKE-UP TRICKS AND TIPS

☆ *Bring a little sparkle to arms and shoulders by mixing a tiny bit of pearlized face powder into your body lotion.*

☆ *If you're having a facial, make sure it's at least a week prior to the wedding. Facials can be detoxing on the skin, resulting in blemishes.*

☆ *A silvery white shadow brushed across the eyes makes the whites of the eyes look even whiter and is a fabulous look for blondes and those with baby-blue eyes.*

☆ *Face shine is your number one enemy in pictures. Make sure you have a compact of ultra-light powder in your bag so you can give yourself a light dusting before smiling for the camera.*

☆ *Avoid lip gloss if you're wearing a veil—it will stick to your lips. Instead, use a dab of petroleum jelly.*

do's and don't's before your wedding day

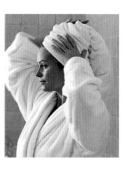
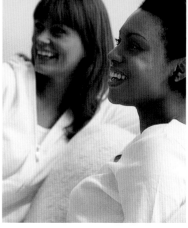

THE NIGHT BEFORE

• Don't drink large amounts of alcohol. It will dehydrate you, encourage a hangover, and won't make you look or feel good on the big day.

• Do spend time with people who relax you.

• Don't eat gas-causing foods like beans, broccoli, and cauliflower. They can all cause bloating.

• Do check buttons and zippers on your gown. And hang the dress out of harm's way!

• Don't take sleeping pills. You'll feel groggy the next morning. Go for herbal tea or warm milk instead.

• Do get some beauty sleep. A few drops of lavender essential oil on your pillow equals restful sleep. If possible, sleep on your back. It lessens the risk of crease lines on your face and décolletage.

• Do make a timetable for getting ready, and stick to it!

• Don't expect everything to run smoothly. Add in an extra hour (set your alarm) in case of any last-minute glitches, such as a broken nail.

• Do wish your partner luck before bedtime. It's his big day tomorrow too, and he's sure to be feeling nervous!

THE BIG DAY

• Do run an early bath and enjoy time on your own.

• Don't have too many glasses of champagne. You don't want to be burping or slurring your vows!

• Do soak two cotton pads in lukewarm green tea and place them on puffy eyes for 10 minutes. A natural anti-inflammatory, the tea will reduce swelling in the area.

• Don't pick up your bouquet if pollen hasn't been removed from the stamens. It may stain your dress.

• Do compliment your flower girls, bridesmaids, and mother on how beautiful they look.

• Don't panic about creases in your veil. Simply use your hairdryer on a medium setting to remove the wrinkles.

• Do keep your sense of humor and remember that this day is about love and celebration. Relax, smile, and enjoy!

• Don't be embarrassed about shedding a tear or two.

• Do look to a holistic fix to stay calm. Drop Bach's Rescue Remedy onto your tongue just before the ceremony begins—it's the hip way to calm nerves.

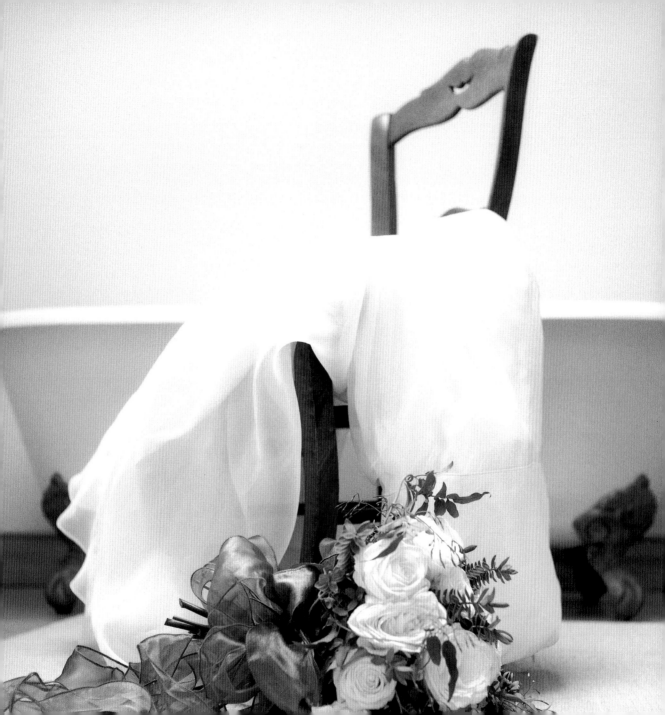

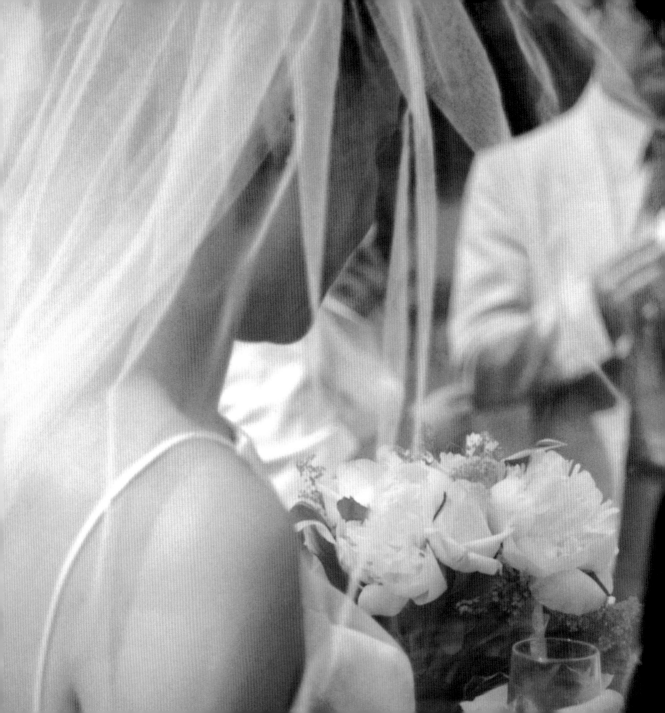

the big day

Months of careful planning have finally come
to an end, and it's your wedding day! Take deep,
meditative breaths to soothe any last-minute
nerves and follow a few essential steps to ensure
your big day goes smoothly.

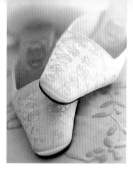

get prepped

THE BASICS Apply deodorant and body lotions as early as possible, so they have time to sink into your skin. You do not want to reveal cakey white armpits, so use a stainless roll-on deodorant. Eat a substantial breakfast and be sure to have more than just a quick coffee. There's nothing worse than the sound of a rumbling tummy during the ceremony, or feeling faint or light-headed because of hunger! Oats have a calming effect, so eat some oatmeal or pancakes. Crank on some relaxing music, and, if your bridesmaids or mother are getting ready with you, make them responsible for minor jobs that will help you keep organized and on schedule.

HAIR AND MAKE-UP Dress in comfortable clothes while you're having your hair and make-up done. Make sure they're easy to remove and don't have to go over your head—the last thing you want to do is mess up your hair! Whether you're doing your make-up yourself or having a professional team do it for you, enjoy the pampering. If you are doing your own make-up, give yourself plenty of time. If your headpiece or veil has pearls on it, spray your hair before fixing it in place (hairspray ruins pearls).

CLEVER DRESSING If your dress is strapless or has a low-back, do not wear a bra on the morning of the wedding, as it can cause skin marks that take hours to fade. When it's time to get dressed, slip on your underwear, bra, stockings, slip, and garter. Now step into

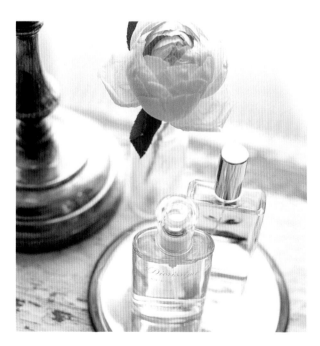

your dress. Allow 15 minutes to slowly fasten and adjust the dress. Zip and button it up little by little to avoid a broken zipper or pulled-off buttons. A long gown needs static protection, so spray a static guard generously. This ensures that the only thing that clings to you is your groom! Put on your shoes, first having gently marked the soles with a knife or scuffed them with a nail file so they are not slippery. Swap your engagement ring to your right hand and put on the rest of your jewelry. When you move, hold a long dress up gently. Clutching it in a sweaty palm will only cause wrinkles.

BAGS OF STYLE You only need somewhere to slip a lipstick and compact, so think lightweight, delicate, and small when it comes to bags. When choosing a bag, make sure it complements the color and the fabric of your dress. Remember that clutch bags need to be carried in your hands, while a small handbag can dangle from the wrist, leaving hands free to meet and greet guests.

BRIDAL EMERGENCY KIT

Be prepared! Put together an emergency kit and give to your maid of honor or a bridesmaid. Include a small sewing kit, tissues, mints, stockings, the nail polish you are wearing (nothing looks worse than a chipped nail), hairbrush, headache tablets, eye drops, and baby powder (useful for any spills on the dress).

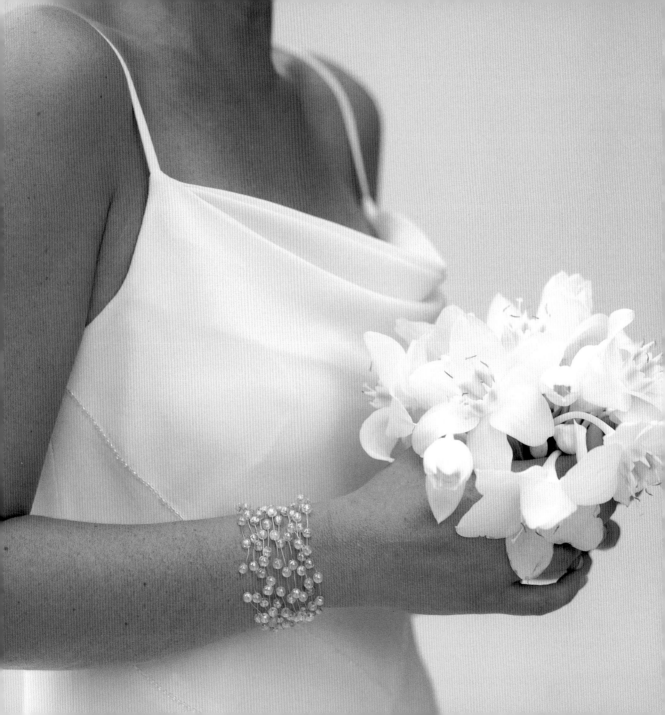

making your entrance

Eye-catching gems and a stunning wedding dress certainly get you noticed, but it's the small details that make for a truly beautiful bride.

POSTURE PERFECT Standing tall tells the world (and your wedding guests) that you feel great about yourself. A few simple techniques are all it takes to look instantly taller and leaner. Straighten your back, drop your shoulders, pull in your stomach, and try to hold this position when walking, standing, and sitting. Control your arms and keep them parallel to the body as much as possible. Finally, lengthen your neck and tilt your chin up for an air of relaxed confidence.

EXITING A CAR GRACEFULLY It's a pretty simple technique. Before the door is opened, straighten your dress and swivel your knees towards the door. When the door is open, swing both legs out at the same time and stand up. The biggest mistake is sticking one leg out, then the other. That's when you risk letting more than your garter show! If you are wearing a wrap, put it on after you exit the car. Don't get out clutching everything; otherwise, you'll look like a bag lady!

GLIDE, DON'T STRIDE Heels add inches to your height. Just make sure you glide in them for maximum effect. The secret to an elegant walk lies in overlapping your feet rather than walking with them side by side. This makes for a clomping walk rather than a graceful effect. Shorten your steps and step with your heel first, then let the sole follow quickly and smoothly. Walk with your toes pointing straight ahead and keep your legs straight, close, and parallel. When it comes to wedding shoes, avoid mules. They're very hard to keep on and walk in elegantly for a long period of time.

LOOKING GOOD IN PHOTOGRAPHS There are rules to follow for giving a good picture. First, practice your pose. Turn your body slightly to the side so you aren't facing the camera straight on, place one foot in front of the other, move your chest and neck forwards, and stick your bottom out slightly. This will elongate and angle your body wonderfully. To avoid a double chin, lift your head up slightly and angle it to the side to define your bone structure. If you find yourself squinting move out of the sun, and if you have silver fillings don't throw your head back and laugh!

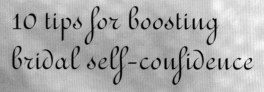

10 tips for boosting bridal self-confidence

You look fabulous—now you want to feel it! For sky-high confidence, lighten your emotional load and look to ways of boosting your self-esteem.

1 If you're feeling nervous, focus on love. It sounds corny, but when you think of someone you really love (like your soon-to-be-husband!), you can't really experience nerves at the same time.

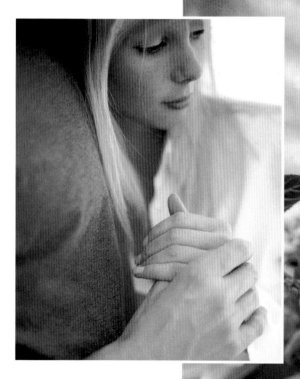

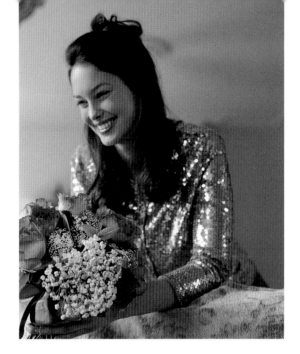

2 Maintain good eye contact when you're exchanging vows with your partner. It helps you feel strong, lays nerves to rest, and shows that you feel confident and believe in what you're saying.

3 Remember to touch your partner. With all the attention and people vying for your attention, it can be easy to lose sight (as well as touch) of each other. Take time to hold hands and give each other little kisses when the camera and eyes are off you. Not only does touch release feel-good chemicals, it revitalizes you, too.

4 If you feel tension building up, shake your arms and legs loosely for a few minutes. The physical movement releases stress, and the spontaneity is freeing.

5 Think yourself fabulous... because you are! Positive thinking can help your mind get to where you want it to be. Shake off any last-minute doubts and stresses by saying to yourself "I look gorgeous!"

6 Give compliments graciously throughout the day. There is no greater confidence than making someone else feel great about themselves, too.

7 Speak up and keep your voice strong and clear. Your voice reveals your emotions, so a joyful and confident tone will say it all.

8 Be friendly with everyone at the reception. There's often an undercurrent of family tension at large gatherings, so choose to ignore it and delight in the fact that everybody is celebrating for you. This action will make your day even more special.

9 Have fun. It's a party! The more laid-back and care-free you are, the more confident you become.

10 Remind yourself that you're getting a loving partner for life. What could be a bigger confidence boost?

sources

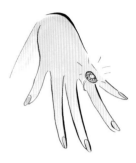

NUTRITION & FITNESS

Fitness Together
www.fitnesstogether.com
Personal-training studios located nationwide. You'll receive one-on-one fitness instruction and a program will be designed to suit your specific needs.

InVite Health
800-844-9060
www.invitehealth.com
Nutritional boutiques in the New York metro area. Accredited nutritionists offer free health- and diet-related advice.

SKINCARE

American Academy of Dermatology
888-462-DERM
www.aad.org

Find a dermatologist in your area through the site's extensive network of physicians.

Clarins
www.clarins.com
Skincare products, facial treatments, and skincare advice are available at retail stores.

Philosophy
800-568-3151
www.philosophy.com
Try their cute "Here Comes the Bride" kit.

EYEBROWS

Anastasia Beverly Hills
www.anastasia.net
Eyebrow guru Anastasia Soare counts Madonna and Jennifer Lopez among her clients. Brow waxing, tweezing, and tinting are available at her two salons in California as well as select Nordstrom and Sephora stores.

Natasha Style & Cut
2759 West Devon Avenue
Chicago, IL 60659
773-761-2274
Salon owner Bharati Nakum is well-known for her threading technique, an ancient form of eyebrow shaping.

HAIR AND MAKEUP

Benefit
800-781-2336
www.benefitcosmetics.com
Check out the brand's "Fake-it" collection to help you get gorgeous for your big day.

Bobbi Brown
877-310-9222
www.bobbibrowncosmetics.com
Request a bridal consultation at any of the Bobbi Brown counters, and you'll receive a free personalized makeup lesson.

Estée Lauder
877-311-3883
www.esteelauder.com
The website has a bridal section. You can also set up a consultation with a beauty advisor at an Estée Lauder counter.

Lips & Locks
642 A. Venice Blvd.
Venice, CA 90291
310-301-8086
www.lipsandlocks.com
A hair and makeup studio helmed by celebrity stylist Sheree Pouls. Bridal consultations include full run-throughs of

hairstyles and makeup combinations.

ModelBride
276 Fifth Avenue
New York, NY 10001
and
240 Main Street
Chatham, NJ 07928
866-900-0456
www.modelbride.com
Makeup artist Lori Dunn and her staff will bring hair and makeup services to your home.

PAMPERING AND TANNING

Canyon Ranch SpaClubs
At The Venetian
3355 Las Vegas Boulevard South, Suite 1159
Las Vegas, NV 89109
877-220-2688
and
At the Gaylord Palms Resort & Convention Center
6000 W. Osceola Parkway
Kissimmee, FL 34746
407-586-2051
www.canyonranch.com
Hair and makeup, manicures, pedicures, massages, facials, wraps, and body scrubs.

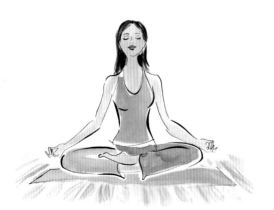

Fantasy Tan
888-FAN-TANS
www.fantasytan.com
Airbrush and spray tans. Visit the
website for your nearest salon.

mobileSPA
800-651-4740
www.mobilespa.com
Spa services and themed spa
parties at home.

Red Mountain Spa
1275 E. Red Mountain Circle
Ivins, UT 84738
800-407-3002
www.redmountainspa.com
Their "Girlfriends Getaway"
package is designed especially
for a bride and her maids.

SPARTY!
646-736-1777
www.spa-party.com
Spa services and parties at home.
Available in major metropolitan
areas.

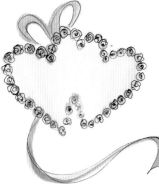

St. Tropez Tanning
661-775-6900
www.sttropeztan.com
The original fake-tan experts.
Visit the website to find your
nearest salon.

FRAGRANCE

The Fragrance Shop Perfumery
612 Lincoln Road
Miami Beach, FL 33139
305-535-0037
www.thefragranceshop.com
Pure perfume oils inspired by
designer fragrances, in addition
to a range of house blends.

WEDDING GOWNS

David's Bridal
877-923-BRIDE
www.davidsbridal.com
Dresses by designers like Oleg
Cassini, veils, shoes, and more.

Designer Loft
226 West 37th Street, 15th Floor
New York, NY 10018
212-944-9013
www.designerloftnyc.com
Gowns by Atelier Aimée and
Manalé. and bridal accessories.

House of Brides
800-395-1240
www.theweddingdresses.com
Online bridal boutique selling
gowns by Alfred Angelo, Paula
Varsalona, Watters & Watters,
and many others. Bridesmaid
dresses, flower-girl
dresses, and accessories
also available.

J. Crew
800-562-0258
www.jcrew.com
Simple and sophisticated
wedding collections, including
bridesmaid dresses, shoes,
jewelry, and handbags.

Monique Lhuillier
www.moniquelhuillier.com
Her modern yet romantic dresses
are available at her salons in
Beverly Hills and Minneapolis, as
well as high-end boutiques and
department stores.

Vera Wang
www.verawang.com
Wang's innovative gowns have
made her a household name.
Visit the website for your
nearest stockist.

WEDDING SHOES

Bellissima Bridal Shoes
866-900-0456
www.bellissimabridalshoes.com
Shoes by designers like Vera
Wang and Cynthia Rowley.

BRIDAL LINGERIE

Agent Provocateur
www.agentprovocateur.com
Wedding lingerie as well as saucy
little numbers for the honeymoon!

La Petite Coquette
888-473-5799
www.thelittleflirt.net
Shop online for "Just Married"
cotton thongs and sheer
babydoll chemises.

Victoria's Secret
800-411-5116
www.victoriassecret.com
Nationwide chain offering a
variety of seamless, strapless,
and push-up bras that will
help you look fabulous in your
gown. Visit the website for
details of your nearest store.

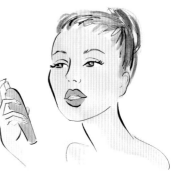

WEDDING PLANNERS

David Tutera
914-777-3817
www.davidtutera.com
New York-based event designer.

Mindy Weiss
800-777-3414
www.mindyweiss.com
An event planner who has
designed both large-scale and
intimate weddings for a slew
of celebrities.

picture credits

Key: a=above, b=below, r=right, l=left, c=center.

All illustrations by Robyn Neilb. All photographs by Winfried Heinze, unless otherwise stated.

Daniel Farmer: pages 19a, 24, 37al, 37br, 50c, 50r, 51l, 51c, 52 both. Claire Richardson: endpapers, pages 28, 34, 44, 45, 46l, 46c, 47, 56l. Dan Duchars: pages 5ar both, 23b, 26l, 27b, 29r, 38l, 50l, 54. Craig Fordham: pages 1, 2, 3, 5l, 7, 20, 30l, 40, 53, 60r, 61. Polly Wreford: pages 4, 31l, 38r, 46r, 56r, 57, 58, 60l. David Montgomery: pages 19b, 25, 29l, 33ar, 36, 39b, 59. Chris Everard: pages 8, 26r. Caroline Arber: page48. Nicki Dowey: page 22r. Andrew Wood: page 37ar.

acknowledgements

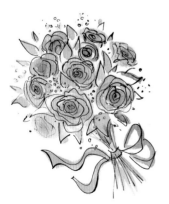

My own wedding was very small, but very beautiful. Whatever type of wedding you choose, a bride always needs to feel special, so I dedicate this book to my two friends Carolyn and Clive Boyland, who helped to organize my wedding day and made me feel just that.

This book is a collection of insiders' tips passed on to me through interviewing many experts in the beauty and fashion industry. There are so many people I would like to thank, but special thanks must go to Michelle Marsh and Ariane Poole for their invaluable make-up tips, Wendy Carrig for her brilliant photographic insights, Janet Ginnings for her colonic cleanser recipe, Kate Cook for her advice on nutrition, and Sarah Maxwell, a wonderful personal trainer, for her exercise tips.

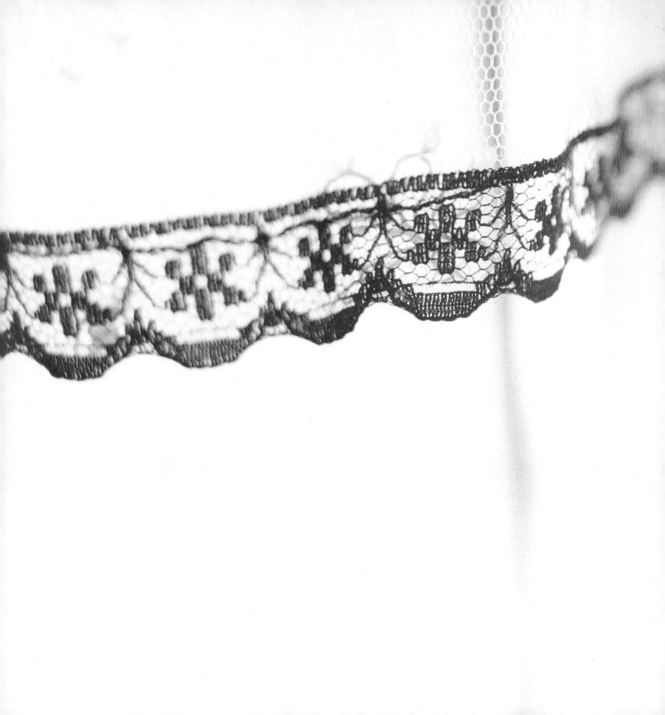